26 Healthy Kid-Friendly Recipes on a Budget

by Kendall Raines

Table of Contents

1. Oatmeal Blueberry Squares

Prep and cook time: 25 minutes

What you need:

- 1½ cups quick oats
- ½ cup whole-wheat flour
- ½ teaspoon baking soda
- ½ teaspoon salt
- 1 teaspoon cinnamon
- ½ cup fresh or frozen blueberries
- 1 egg
- 1 cup skim milk
- 3 tablespoons apple sauce
- ¼ cup brown sugar

Equipment and supplies:

- Large mixing bowl
- 8x8-inch baking pan
- Measuring cups and spoons

What to do:

1. Preheat oven to 350° F.
2. Coat baking pan with cooking spray.
3. Place all of the ingredients into a large bowl and mix until just combined.
4. Pour into prepared pan and bake for 20 minutes or until a toothpick inserted into the center comes out clean.
5. Allow to cool for 5 minutes and cut into squares.

How much does this recipe make?
9 squares

2. Fun Pizza for Kids

Prep time: 90 minutes

What you need:

For the cauliflower crusts

- 1 medium head cauliflower, chopped
- 1 cup shredded part-skim mozzarella cheese
- 1 large egg
- ½ teaspoon garlic powder
- ½ teaspoon dried oregano
- ¼ teaspoon salt

For the pizza topping

- ½ pound lean ground beef
- ¼ cup shredded yellow squash
- ¼ cup shredded zucchini
- 1 clove garlic, minced
- ¼ teaspoon dried oregano
- Freshly ground black pepper (to taste)
- ½ cup tomato sauce
- 1 cup shredded part-skim mozzarella cheese

Optional toppings

- 16 cherry tomatoes (halved)
- 3 tablespoons sliced almonds
- ½ cup chopped broccoli florets
- ½ cup sliced mushrooms
- Several leaves of baby spinach

Equipment and supplies:

- Measuring cups and spoons

- Food processor
- Baking sheet lined with parchment paper
- Knife for chopping
- Kitchen towel
- Medium bowl
- Spoon for stirring
- Microwave
- Sauté pan

What to do:

Make the cauliflower crusts:

1. Preheat the oven to 400°F (204°C).
2. Line a large baking sheet with parchment paper.
3. In a food processor, pulse the cauliflower into very small pieces.
4. Transfer to a microwave-safe bowl and microwave until tender, about 4 minutes. Let the cauliflower cool for several minutes.
5. Wrap the cooled cauliflower in a kitchen towel and squeeze out any excess liquid.
6. In a medium bowl, combine the cauliflower, mozzarella cheese, egg, garlic powder, oregano, and salt.
7. Stir to combine.
8. Divide the mixture into 8 equal parts and form each one into a ball.
9. Press and flatten the balls into circles or fun shapes.
10. Place them onto the prepared baking sheet.
11. Bake the pizza crusts for 15 minutes.
12. Flip crusts over and continue baking for another 15 minutes, until firm and light golden brown.
13. Remove the crusts from the oven, but leave the oven on.

While crusts are baking, make the toppings:

1. In a large sauté pan over moderate heat, cook the ground beef, yellow squash, zucchini, garlic, oregano, and pepper.

2. Stir to break up the beef and continue cooking until the beef is cooked through, about 8 minutes. Drain any excess liquid.

Assemble and bake the pizzas:

1. Spread the tomato sauce on the crusts.
2. Top the pizzas with the beef mixture, cheese, and any optional toppings you choose.
3. Bake until the cheese bubbles, about 6 minutes. (For a delicious smoky taste, heat pizzas on a wood-fire or charcoal grill.)

How much does this recipe make?

4 servings / 2 mini pizzas per person

3. Confetti Soup

Prep time: 1 hour

What you need:

- 2 teaspoons canola oil
- 2 cups raw carrots, diced
- 1/3 cup raw kale, chopped
- ¼ cup onion, chopped
- ¼ cup celery, chopped
- ½ teaspoon black pepper
- 3½ cups water
- 2 tablespoons raw parsley
- ¼ teaspoon whole fennel seed
- Pinch of crushed red pepper
- 1 pound black-eyed peas
- ½ pound turkey ham
- ½ teaspoon salt

Equipment and Supplies

- Strainer
- Large stockpot
- Measuring cups/spoons
- Oven/stove

What to do:

1. Place a large pot over medium high heat. Add the oil, chopped onion, and chopped celery and cook until translucent (the pieces will be soft and you can sort of see through them).
2. Add the diced carrots, salt, pepper, fennel seed, and crushed red pepper. Cook for 2-3 minutes.

3. Add the black-eyed peas and water and cook for 25-30 minutes.
4. When the peas are soft, add the turkey ham and kale and cook for another 10 minutes until the kale is tender.
5. Adjust seasoning (if necessary) and serve.

How much does this recipe make?
Six servings

4. Yummy Oatmeal

Prep time: about 10 minutes

Ingredients:

- 1 c. water
- ½ c. rolled oats
- dash of salt
- ¼ c. applesauce
- pinch of cinnamon
- 2 tsp. brown sugar

Utensils:

- cooking pot
- measuring cups and spoons
- stove (you'll need help from your adult assistant)
- mixing spoon
- serving bowl

Directions:

1. Pour the water, oats, and salt into a medium-size pot on the stovetop.
2. Heat the mixture until it boils, then turn the heat to low.
3. Using a wooden spoon, stir in the applesauce and cinnamon.
4. Cook on low heat and continue to stir the mixture for 5 minutes.
5. Pour the oatmeal into a bowl and sprinkle the brown sugar on top.
6. Allow the oatmeal to cool for a minute before digging in.

Serves: 1

Serving size: 1 bowl

Nutritional analysis (per serving):
390 calories
13 g protein
6 g fat
74 g carbohydrate
9 g fiber
0 mg cholesterol
302 mg sodium
64 mg calcium
4.3 mg iron

5. Satisfying Strawberry Bars

Prep time: 45 minutes

Ingredients:

- 1 c. flour
- 1 c. rolled oats
- ½ c. butter or margarine, softened
- 1/3 c. light brown sugar
- ¼ tsp. baking powder
- 1/8 tsp. salt
- ¾ c. strawberry jam

Utensils:

- oven (you'll need help from your adult assistant)
- large bowl
- square (8" x 8") pan coated with nonstick spray
- large spoon
- knife (you'll need help from your adult assistant)
- measuring cups and spoons

Directions:

1. Preheat oven to 350° Fahrenheit (180° Celsius).
2. In a large bowl, mix everything together except the strawberry jam.
3. Measure out 2 cups of this mixture. Leave the rest in the bowl, and set it aside.
4. Take the 2 cups of the mixture and press it into the bottom of the pan. You can use your hands or a spoon. Make sure you cover the entire bottom of the pan!
5. Using a large spoon, spread the strawberry jam on top of the mixture in the pan. Spread it evenly all over.
6. Take the mixture that was left in the bowl, and spread it over the strawberry jam. Press it down lightly.

7. Bake for 25 minutes. Remove the pan from the oven, and allow it to cool for at least 15 minutes.
8. Cut the bars into 12 squares to eat and share!

Serves: 12

Serving size: 1 square

6. Almond, Cocoa, & Oat Clusters

Prep time: 25 minutes

What you need:

- 2 cups rolled oats
- ¼ cup fat-free milk
- 4 tablespoons yogurt spread (also can use vegetable oil spread)
- 1/3 cup brown sugar
- 2 tablespoons unsweetened cocoa powder
- ¼ cup smooth, unsalted almond butter (or other nut or soy butter)
- ½ teaspoon vanilla extract
- 1/3 cup raisins

Equipment and supplies:

- Baking sheet
- Wax paper
- Large mixing bowl
- Medium saucepan
- Measuring spoons

What to do:

1. Line a baking sheet with wax paper and set aside.
2. Place oats into a large bowl.
3. In a medium saucepan, heat milk and yogurt spread over medium heat.
4. When the spread is melted, whisk in brown sugar and cocoa powder.
5. Keep stirring while you bring the mixture to a boil.

6. Turn down the heat and continue cooking the sauce for 1 minute.
7. Remove the pan from the heat and stir in almond butter, vanilla extract, and raisins.
8. Immediately pour the sauce over the rolled oats and stir well until oats are completely covered in sauce.
9. Place rounded tablespoon-size scoops of the mixture onto prepared baking sheet.
10. Allow clusters to set for 15 minutes before serving.

How much does this recipe make?

12 cookies

7. Hawaiin Kids Turkey Sliders

Prep time: 30 minutes

What you need:

For the mango-pineapple salsa:

- 1 ripe mango, peeled and diced
- 1 cup diced fresh (or canned in juice) pineapple
- 1 to 2 small jalapeños, finely diced (optional)
- 3 tablespoons diced Bermuda or Vidalia onion
- Juice of 1 medium lime
- Pinch of sea salt
- Freshly ground black pepper

For the Hawaiian turkey sliders:

- 2 pounds ground turkey
- 1 clove garlic, peeled and crushed
- 3 tablespoons ketchup
- 1 tablespoon extra-virgin olive oil
- 1 tablespoon gluten-free soy sauce
- 1 tablespoon dried cilantro
- 1 teaspoon onion powder
- ½ teaspoon dried oregano
- Dash of salt
- ¼ teaspoon freshly ground black pepper
- 12 romaine or Bibb lettuce leaves
- 12 gluten-free rolls or whole-grain dinner rolls

Equipment and supplies:

- Medium bowl
- Refrigerator

- Large bowl
- Grill

What to do:

Make the mango-pineapple salsa:

1. In a medium non-metallic bowl, stir together the mango, pineapple, jalapeños, onion, lime juice, salt, and pepper. Cover and chill in the refrigerator until ready to use. (The salsa is best when made several hours to one day in advance.)

Make the Hawaiian turkey sliders:

1. In a large bowl, combine the turkey, garlic, ketchup, olive oil, soy sauce, cilantro, onion powder, oregano, salt, and pepper. Gently mix the ingredients until they are thoroughly combined.
2. Divide the mixture into 12 equal parts and shape each one into a ball that is slightly smaller than a tennis ball. Using the palm of your hand, gently flatten each into a patty.
3. Heat a grill or barbecue to medium-high heat. Grill the turkey sliders until cooked through, about 5 minutes per side.
4. Place one lettuce leaf on the bottom of each roll. Serve the sliders on the rolls, topped with a dollop of mango-pineapple salsa.

How much does this recipe make? 12 sliders

8. Little Porcupine Sliders

Prep time: 90 minutes

What you need:

- 1/3 cup brown rice, uncooked
- ½ teaspoon salt
- ¾ teaspoon canola oil
- 1½ tablespoons yellow onion, chopped
- 1 medium stalk of celery, finely chopped
- 1 clove garlic, minced
- 1 pound ground turkey, extra lean
- 1 large egg
- 1½ tablespoons dried cranberries
- ¾ cup spinach leaves
- ¾ teaspoon Worcestershire sauce
- ½ teaspoon black pepper
- 1 pinch ground red pepper
- Small wheat rolls

Equipment and supplies

- Measuring cups/spoons
- Knife
- Sheet pans
- Large skillet
- Bowls

What to do:

1. Preheat oven to 350°F.
2. Cook rice according to package directions and include the ½ teaspoon of salt. When done, drain well and spread on a sheet pan to cool completely.

3. Add canola oil to heated skillet. Add onion, celery, and garlic and sauté until soft (about 5 minutes). Transfer to sheet pan with rice and cool completely.
4. In a large mixing bowl, combine turkey, egg, cranberries, spinach, Worcestershire sauce, black pepper, and red pepper. Mix well.
5. Add rice and vegetable mixture to turkey mixture.
6. Form into 6 patties. Place on sheet pan.
7. Bake in preheated oven for 25 minutes until turkey reaches an internal temperature of 165°F.
8. Serve on whole-wheat rolls with optional lettuce, tomato, and red onion.

How much does this recipe make?
Six servings

9. Chicken Chex

Prep time: 50 minutes

What you need:

- 1 cup gluten-free corn cereal, such as Chex
- ¼ cup gluten-free baked veggie chips (chili limon flavor works well)
- ¼ cup pecans
- 1 teaspoon ground lemon pepper
- 3 large egg whites
- 8 ounces boneless, skinless chicken breast, halved
- 1 medium yellow squash, cut into half moons
- 1 medium zucchini, cut into half moons
- ½ cup sliced carrots

Equipment and supplies:

- Oven
- Large bowl
- Small bowl
- Baking dish
- Small saucepan
- Knife

What to do:

1. Preheat the oven to 350°F (176°C).
2. In a large bowl, stir together the cereal, veggie chips, pecans, and lemon pepper. Smash and combine the cereal mixture.
3. Place the egg whites in a small bowl.
4. Working with 1 piece at a time, dip the chicken into the cereal mixture then dip it into the egg whites, then back into the cereal mixture, making sure all of the chicken is covered. Transfer the "breaded" chicken to a baking dish and repeat with the remaining chicken, cereal mixture, and egg whites.

5. Bake the chicken until golden brown, about 30 minutes.
6. While the chicken is baking, bring a small saucepan of water to a boil. Add the squash, zucchini, and carrots and simmer, lowering the heat if necessary, until tender, about 7 minutes. Serve the veggies with the chicken.

How much does this recipe make? 2 servings

10. Tortilla Bowl Delight

What you need:

- 1 medium (4-ounce) boneless, skinless chicken breast, grilled or cooked as desired, and cut into bite-size pieces
- ¼ cup diced avocado
- ¼ cup diced orange bell pepper
- ¼ cup diced tomato
- ¼ cup lactose-free shredded Monterey Jack cheese (can substitute regular cheese if you have no dietary restrictions)
- Salt and freshly ground black pepper
- 1 corn tortilla bowl

Equipment and supplies:

- Medium bowl
- Knife

What to do:

1. In a medium bowl, toss together the chicken, avocado, bell pepper, tomato, and cheese.
2. Season with salt and pepper.
3. Scoop into the tortilla bowl and serve immediately.

How much does this recipe make? 1 tortilla bowl

11. Healthy Kids Garden Chicken Wrap

Prep time: 5-10 minutes

What you need:

- 4 whole-wheat wraps (8 inches)
- 2 cups store-bought rotisserie chicken, shredded
- ½ cup shredded carrots
- 1 avocado, thinly sliced
- 1 cup baby spinach leaves
- ¼ cup of your favorite fat-free/low-fat dressing (about 1 tablespoon per wrap)

Equipment and supplies:

- Cutting board
- Sharp knife
- Measuring cups

What to do:

1. Place wraps side by side on a flat surface. Divide chicken into four portions (about ½ cup each). Place a portion of chicken on each wrap.
2. Top each wrap with carrots, avocado, and spinach. (Have an adult help with the chopping.)
3. Drizzle dressing evenly over each wrap.
4. Roll each wrap up tightly and cut on the diagonal.
5. Serve immediately or wrap tightly in aluminum foil and refrigerate for lunch the next day.

How much does this recipe make?

4 wraps

12. Tots for Tots

Prep time: 1 hour

What you need:

- 1½ pounds sweet potatoes
- ¾ cup chickpeas (also called garbanzo beans), undrained
- 2 tablespoons vegetable oil
- ½ teaspoon salt
- ¼ teaspoon pepper
- ½ teaspoon onion powder
- ½ teaspoon cinnamon
- Cooking spray

Equipment and supplies:

- Measuring cups/spoons
- Knife
- Food processor
- Large bowl
- Sheet pans
- Oven/stove

What to do:

1. Preheat oven to 400°F.
2. Steam or boil sweet potatoes until barely tender, approximately 15 minutes. Let cool.
3. Peel cooled potatoes. Shred them using a grater or food processor.
4. Puree chickpeas, including liquid, until smooth.
5. Combine shredded sweet potatoes and chickpeas in a large bowl.
6. Add oil, salt, pepper, onion powder, and cinnamon. Mix well.
7. Spray sheet pans with cooking spray.

8. Scoop heaping tablespoons of the mixture and place 1 inch apart on prepared sheet pans.
9. Bake in oven for approximately 10-12 minutes, until starting to brown.

How much does this recipe make?
Six servings

13. Half Pint Peanut Butter Muffins

Prep time: 35 minutes

Ingredients:

- 2 eggs
- 1 c. milk
- ¼ c. banana (about 1 banana), mashed with a fork
- ¼ c. peanut butter
- 1/3 c. vegetable oil
- ¼ c. frozen apple juice concentrate, thawed (left out of the freezer until it's soft)
- ¼ c. nonfat dry milk
- 2¼ c. flour
- 1½ tsp. baking powder
- 1 tsp. baking soda
- nonstick cooking spray

Utensils:

- oven (you'll need help from your adult assistant)
- fork
- small bowl
- large bowl
- mixing spoon
- muffin/cupcake tin
- paper muffin/cupcake liners
- wire rack
- measuring cups and spoons

Directions:

1. Preheat oven to 350° F (180° C).

2. In a small bowl, break the eggs and use a fork to beat them a little bit.
3. In a large bowl, combine the milk, mashed banana, peanut butter, vegetable oil, apple juice, dry milk, and the eggs from the small bowl. Mix with a mixing spoon until the mixture is creamy.
4. Add the flour, baking powder, and baking soda into the large bowl. Mix again.
5. Line a muffin tine with paper liners or lightly spray with nonstick spray. Spoon in the muffin mix. Fill each muffin cup about 2/3 of the way up.
6. Bake for about 15 minutes.
7. When your muffins are finished baking, remove from muffin tin and cool them on the wire rack. Then it's time to taste and share!

Serves: 12

Serving size: 1 muffin

14. Fruity Banana Smoothie

Prep time: 15 minutes

What you need:

- 8 passion fruits, seeded and flesh removed
- 4 bananas, peeled
- 2 cups fat-free plain Greek-style yogurt
- 2 tablespoons honey
- 8 ice cubes

Equipment and supplies:

- Measuring cups and spoons
- Knife
- Blender

What to do:

1. In a blender, combine the passion fruits, bananas, yogurt, honey, and ice cubes.
2. Blend until smooth.

How much does this recipe make?

4 servings

15. Yogurt Pineapple Pops

Prep time: about 1-2 hours

Ingredients:

- 2 c. plain yogurt
- ½ c. canned crushed pineapple (packed in its own juice instead of packed in syrup)
- 1 can frozen pineapple or orange-pineapple juice concentrate, thawed

Utensils:

- medium-sized bowl
- mixing spoon
- small paper cups
- plastic wrap
- wooden popsicle sticks (available at craft stores)
- measuring cups

Directions:

1. Drain the can of crushed pineapple so all the juice runs out.
2. Put all the ingredients in the bowl and mix together.
3. Spoon the mixture into the paper cups. Fill them almost to the top.
4. Stretch a small piece of plastic wrap across the top of each cup.
5. Using the popsicle stick, poke a hole in the plastic wrap. Stand the stick straight up in the center of the cup.
6. Put the cups in the freezer until the mixture is frozen solid.
7. Remove the plastic wrap and peel away the paper cup. You'll have pineapple pops to eat and share!

Serves: 6

Serving size: 1 pop

16. Easy On-the-Go Snack Mix

Prep time: 5 minutes

What you need:

- 1 cup whole grain cereal (squares or Os work best)
- ¼ cup dried fruit of your choice
- ¼ cup nuts, such as walnut pieces, slivered almonds, or pistachios
- ¼ cup small, whole-grain snack crackers or pretzels

Equipment and supplies:

- Large bowl
- Measuring cups
- Large spoon

What to do:

1. Measure out ingredients.
2. Combine in large bowl.

How much does this recipe make?

Three to four ½-cup servings

17. Refreshing Fruit Kabobs

Prep time: 15 minutes

Ingredients:

- 1 apple
- 1 banana
- 1/3 c. red seedless grapes
- 1/3 c. green seedless grapes
- 2/3 cup pineapple chunks
- 1 cup nonfat yogurt
- ¼ c. dried coconut, shredded

Utensils:

- knife (you'll need help from your adult assistant)
- 2 wooden skewer sticks
- large plate

Directions:

1. Prepare the fruit by washing the grapes, washing the apples and cutting them into small squares, peeling the bananas and cutting them into chunks, and cutting the pineapple into chunks, if it's fresh. Put the fruit onto a large plate.
2. Spread coconut onto another large plate.
3. Slide pieces of fruit onto the skewer and design your own kabob by putting as much or as little of whatever fruit you want! Do this until the stick is almost covered from end to end.
4. Hold your kabob at the ends and roll it in the yogurt, so the fruit gets covered. Then roll it in the coconut.
5. Repeat these steps with another skewer.

Serves: 4

18. Homemade Peanut Butter

Prep time: about 10 minutes

Ingredients:

- 1½ c. unsalted roasted peanuts
- 1 tbsp. peanut oil

Utensils:

- food processor (you'll need help from your adult assistant)
- bowl
- mixing spoon
- storage container
- measuring cups and spoons

Directions:

For **smooth** peanut butter:

1. Mix the peanuts with the peanut oil, and pour the mixture into the food processor.
2. Process the mixture until it's very smooth.
3. Store your smooth peanut butter in a sealed container in the fridge. It will be good for 2 weeks.

For **chunky** peanut butter:

1. Take about ¼ cup out of your 1½ cups of peanuts and set them aside.
2. Mix the rest of the peanuts with the oil, and pour the mixture into the food processor.
3. Process the mixture until it's very smooth, then stir in the peanuts that you had set aside.
4. Process a few seconds more to create the chunks in your chunky peanut butter.

5. Store your chunky peanut butter in a sealed container in the fridge. It will be good for 2 weeks.

Serves: 12

Serving size: 2 tablespoons

19. Itzy Bitzy Pizzas For Kids

Prep time: about 15 minutes

Ingredients:

- 1 standard-sized bagel, cut in half
- tomato sauce
- shredded mozzarella cheese
- toppings like diced green pepper, chopped onion, or chopped tomato (whatever you like)
- seasonings like oregano, basil, and pepper

Utensils:

- oven (you'll need help from your adult assistant)
- knife (you'll need help from your adult assistant)
- baking sheet

Directions:

1. Preheat the oven to 325° F.
2. Spread tomato sauce on each bagel half.
3. Sprinkle the shredded cheese all over the tomato sauce on each half.
4. Add your favorite toppings.
5. Put a light sprinkling of seasonings on each half.
6. Put your bagel halves on the baking sheet.
7. Bake in the oven on low heat for about 5 to 8 minutes. You'll know they're done when the cheese is bubbly.
8. Let cool for a minute, then enjoy your tiny pizzas!

Serves: 1

Serving size: 2 tiny pizzas

20. Cheesy Cream Cucumber Sandwich

Prep time: 5-10 minutes

What you need:

- ¾ cup light cream cheese, slightly softened
- half a large cucumber, thinly sliced
- 8 slices of whole-wheat bread

Equipment and supplies:

- Large knife
- Cutting board
- Plastic wrap (optional)

What to do:

1. Spread each slice of bread with cream cheese (about 3 tablespoons per sandwich).
2. Place about 4 cucumber slices on 4 of the slices of bread and top with remaining bread slices.
3. Cut into quarters and serve immediately or wrap sandwiches and save for later.

How much does this make?

4 sandwiches

21. Great Blueberry Pancakes

Prep time: about 20 minutes

Ingredients:

- ¾ c. flour
- 1 tbsp. sugar
- 1 tsp. baking powder
- ½ tsp. salt
- 1 tbsp. margarine
- 1 egg
- ¾ c. milk
- ½ c. blueberries, washed and drained
- extra margarine for the pan

Utensils:

- stove (you'll need help from your adult assistant)
- large bowl
- mixing spoon
- saucepan
- medium-size bowl
- whisk
- measuring cups and spoons
- spatula

Directions:

1. In a large bowl, sift together the flour, sugar, baking powder, and salt. Set the bowl aside.
2. Melt the margarine in a small saucepan.
3. Crack the egg into a medium-size bowl, then add the milk and melted margarine.
4. Whisk egg mixture until it is well mixed.

5. Add the flour mixture to the egg mixture. Whisk again until both mixtures are blended together.
6. Put extra margarine in the saucepan and heat it on the stovetop on medium heat. It is hot enough when the margarine starts to bubble.
7. Use a measuring cup or a small ladle to spoon the batter into the pan. Put some blueberries on top of each pancake.
8. Cook your pancakes on medium heat until small bubbles appear on the top.
9. Use a spatula to see when your pancakes are light brown on the bottom. When they are, flip them over with the spatula.
10. Cook for another few minutes until the pancakes are light brown on the other side.
11. Remove your pancakes and put them on plates to enjoy!

Serves: 2

Serving size: 3 or 4 medium pancakes

22. Friendly Harvest Bake

Prep time: 90 minutes

What you need:

- 1¼ pounds butternut squash, cubed
- 1½ tablespoons red bell pepper, chopped
- 1¾ teaspoon jalapeño pepper, chopped
- 2½ tablespoons yellow onion, diced
- 5 tablespoons applesauce
- 5 tablespoons black beans, drained
- 3½ teaspoons fresh oregano
- 1/8 teaspoon kosher salt
- 3 tablespoons extra virgin olive oil
- 2 tablespoons red quinoa (to be prepared according to package directions)
- ½ cup low-fat granola

Equipment and supplies:

- Knife
- Cutting board
- Sheet pans
- Aluminum foil
- Measuring cups/spoons
- Pot for cooking quinoa
- Three large bowls
- 6x6-inch baking dish
- Oven/stove

What to do:

1. Line two pans with foil.
2. Preheat oven to 350°F.

3. Combine cubed squash, chopped red pepper, and chopped jalapeño pepper in a mixing bowl. Toss with 2 tablespoons olive oil.
4. Place squash mixture on a lined pan and roast in oven for 20 minutes.
5. In a separate bowl, toss chopped onion with 1 tablespoon olive oil.
6. Spread onions on second lined pan and roast in oven for 10 minutes.
7. While vegetables are roasting, prepare 2 tablespoons quinoa according to package directions. Set aside.
8. In large bowl, combine quinoa, applesauce, black beans, oregano, and salt.
9. When cool, add squash mixture and onions to the bowl. Toss lightly.
10. Place into the baking dish.
11. Top with granola.
12. Bake in oven for 20 minutes, or until granola is slightly browned.

How much does this recipe make?

Six ½-cup servings

23. Sloppy Joe with Turkey

Ingredients

- 1 tablespoon(s) olive oil
- 4 carrots, coarsely grated (2 cups)
- 1 medium onion, minced
- 1 clove(s) garlic, minced
- Coarse salt and ground pepper
- 3 tablespoon(s) tomato paste
- 3/4 pound(s) ground turkey (93% lean, dark meat)
- 1 can(s) (28 ounces) crushed tomatoes
- 2 tablespoon(s) dark-brown sugar
- 1 tablespoon(s) cider vinegar
- 1 teaspoon(s) Worcestershire sauce

4 whole-wheat hamburger rolls, split

Directions

1. In a large saucepan, heat oil over medium; add carrots, onion, and garlic. Season with salt and pepper. Cook, stirring occasionally, until softened, 4 to 5 minutes.
2. Add tomato paste and cook, stirring, 1 minute. Add turkey; cook, breaking up meat with a spoon, until no longer pink, 4 to 5 minutes.

Add tomatoes, sugar, vinegar, and Worcestershire sauce. Cook, *stirring occasionally*, until slightly thickened, 12 to 14 minutes. Serve on whole-wheat rolls.

24. Little Hand Chicken Fingers

Yields 3-5 servings
Oven Temperature 375

Ingredients

Chicken Fingers:

- 1 pound(s) chicken tenders (The package might call them "loins")
- 1 cup(s) flour
- 1 teaspoon(s) salt
- 1/2 teaspoon(s) pepper
- 1/4 teaspoon(s) baking powder
- 1 egg
- Cooking spray

Honey Baby Sauce:

- 1/4 cup(s) honey
1/4 cup(s) spicy brown mustard

Directions

1. Preheat the toaster oven to 375 degrees. Rinse the chicken under running water in the colander, and blot it dry with the paper towels. The drying part is important because the coating won't stick to wet chicken, so don't skip it.
2. Combine the dry ingredients in one of the shallow dishes. (Since this recipe uses baking powder, you need to measure out the dry ingredients carefully.) Use the fork to mix them together.

3. Use the fork to beat the egg lightly in the other shallow dish. Now the fun part: dredge each piece of chicken first in the flour (shake off any extra), then in the egg, and then back in the flour. Finally, place the chicken on the baking sheet. Lightly spray the tops of the dredged chicken with oil.
4. Bake for 15 minutes. Flip the chicken pieces over with the tongs. Lightly spray them with oil, and bake another 5 minutes until golden brown.
5. **To make sauce:** Combine honey and mustard in a small bowl. If you're sharing, let each person have their own little bowl of sauce.

Let the chicken fingers cool before you dip them in Honey Baby Sauce. **Chow down.**

25. Children with Diabetes

What is Diabetes?

Diabetes, known in the medical community as diabetes mellitus, is a disorder that makes it difficult for the body to regulate blood sugar levels. Diabetes mellitus occurs in the body's immune system, preventing it from effectively warding off from viruses, bacteria and other foreign substances. Diabetes can be associated with major complications involving many organs including the heart, eyes, kidneys and nerves, especially if the blood sugar is poorly controlled over the years. There are two major types of diabetes: type 1 diabetes and type 2 diabetes.

What is Childhood Diabetes?

Type 1 diabetes, also called juvenile diabetes or insulin-dependent diabetes, occurs when the body's immune system attacks and destroys certain cells in the pancreas, an organ about the size of a hand that is located behind the lower part of the stomach. These cells normally produce insulin, which helps the body move the sugar contained in food into cells throughout the body to provide energy. But when these cells are destroyed, insulin can't be produced, and sugar stays in the blood instead. If left untreated, diabetes can cause serious damage to all the organ systems of the body. Type 1 diabetes can occur at any age, but it most often occurs in children and young adults.

We have put together a unique cookbook for children that are diabetics. If your child has diabetes or maybe prone to this disease, make **SURE** to get our cookbook for diabetics!

www.ingramcontent.com/pod-product-compliance
Lightning Source LLC
Chambersburg PA
CBHW071144280526
45787CB00003B/1394